UNDERSTANDING

SHIATSU

TECHNIQUES

FOR BEGINNERS

A Step-By-Step Approach To Applying Shiatsu For Stress Reduction, Muscle Recovery, And Energy Balancing

DR. ALICIA SONYA

CONTENTS

DISCLAIMER

The information provided in this book is for educational and informational purposes only and is not intended as medical advice, diagnosis, or treatment. Always consult with a qualified healthcare professional before beginning any therapy, practice, or lifestyle change.

The author and publisher of this book make no representations or warranties regarding the accuracy, applicability, or completeness of the content presented. While every effort has been made to ensure the information provided is accurate and up-to-date, the field of health and wellness is constantly evolving, and the reader is advised to use discretion and seek professional guidance as needed.

This book contains references to individuals, products, websites, organizations, or other entities solely for informational purposes. The author and publisher do not endorse, sponsor, or affiliate with any of these references, nor do they receive any benefit from their inclusion. The mention of any names, trademarks, or products does not imply any association or endorsement.

The use of this book is solely at the reader's discretion. Neither the author nor the publisher shall be held liable for any damages, loss, or injury resulting from the use or misuse of the information contained herein.

ABOUT THIS BOOK

Understanding Shiatsu Techniques For Beginners offers a comprehensive journey into the art and science of Shiatsu, a Japanese healing method that emphasizes the balancing of energy and relief from physical and mental stress. This guide begins with an insightful introduction to Shiatsu's origins and its roots in traditional Japanese practices. It highlights the profound benefits Shiatsu offers, from alleviating tension and promoting muscle recovery to restoring energy balance throughout the body. Readers are introduced to essential concepts, such as the flow of energy along meridian lines and the importance of pressure points, fostering a deep understanding of how Shiatsu works with the body's natural energies. Practical advice on safety and contraindications ensures that both beginners and practitioners understand when Shiatsu is most beneficial and how to safely apply it.

Creating the right environment is a vital aspect of an effective Shiatsu session, and this guide delves into how to prepare a serene and comfortable space, from selecting suitable mats and tools to employing grounding techniques that benefit the practitioner. Readers are walked through best practices for self-care and hygiene and provided with guidance on how to mentally and physically prepare a recipient for their Shiatsu experience, ensuring each session is both calming and effective.

For those new to Shiatsu, this book introduces foundational techniques, explaining how to use finger pressure and body-weight methods to stimulate energy points effectively. Readers will learn how to apply sustained pressure using the palms, thumbs, and elbows, seamlessly moving between areas to create smooth energy transitions. These simple yet effective methods serve as a gateway for beginners to harness Shiatsu's healing potential.

With a dedicated focus on stress reduction, this guide highlights specific pressure points to calm the nervous system, relieving tension in areas like the shoulders and neck. Readers gain access to gentle, step-by-step sequences designed to promote relaxation and create a peaceful atmosphere conducive to stress relief. This book also explores Shiatsu's value for muscle recovery, guiding readers to identify pain points and use techniques that stimulate circulation and ease muscle soreness. Practical examples provide clear steps for effective recovery sessions, including self-Shiatsu methods for ongoing maintenance and relief.

A core element of Shiatsu is energy balancing, and this guide explains the intricate network of energy meridians and methods for boosting vitality. Readers will discover key points along these meridians, as well as tailored routines to enhance energy levels in the morning and rebalance them at the day's end.

Additionally, this book addresses common ailments like headaches, lower back pain, and digestive discomfort with targeted techniques that can improve sleep and alleviate fatigue.

To foster self-care, the book includes an entire section dedicated to self-Shiatsu, with techniques accessible to anyone for reducing daily stress and enhancing personal wellness. Morning and evening routines are outlined for convenient self-care, along with tips on precautions to observe for safe practice. Common concerns and frequently asked questions are thoroughly addressed, from how often Shiatsu can be practiced to tips on managing post-session soreness, making this guide an accessible reference for users of all backgrounds.

Finally, this book encourages readers to view Shiatsu as an evolving journey. Practical advice on continuing to develop skills, avoiding common mistakes, and practicing on various body types aids practitioners in honing their expertise. Connecting with the broader Shiatsu community and finding additional resources supports ongoing growth, ensuring that readers can deepen their understanding and proficiency in this timeless healing art. This comprehensive guide is not only a resource for mastering Shiatsu but also an invitation to embrace it as a lifelong practice.

CHAPTER ONE

Introduction To Shiatsu

Shiatsu is a traditional Japanese bodywork therapy that uses finger, thumb, and palm pressure along with stretches and joint rotations to improve energy flow and overall well-being. It is based on the same principles as acupuncture, focusing on balancing the body's energy or "Qi" along meridian lines—specific pathways that connect different organs and systems. Practitioners believe that by stimulating these meridian points, they can release blockages and restore natural energy flow, enhancing both physical and mental health.

During a typical Shiatsu session, practitioners work on the entire body, applying pressure to meridian points along the back, arms, legs, and abdomen. Sessions usually begin with gentle rocking or stretching to relax muscles and prepare the body, followed by rhythmic pressing and holding at different points.

Unlike Western massages, Shiatsu is performed on a mat or futon on the floor, with the recipient fully clothed to encourage ease of movement and a focus on energy flow.

For beginners, understanding the holistic nature of Shiatsu is key. Practitioners view the body, mind, and energy as interconnected, aiming not only for physical relief but also for emotional and spiritual balance. Shiatsu is rooted in awareness, so both the practitioner and receiver work together in a state of mindfulness and breathing harmony, enhancing the therapeutic experience.

Overview Of Shiatsu And Its Japanese Origins

Shiatsu evolved from Anma, a traditional Japanese massage method, and has been influenced by both Chinese medicine and Western practices. "Shiatsu" literally means "finger pressure," and the practice became formalized in Japan in the early 20th century. Japanese physician Tokujiro Namikoshi developed and popularized modern Shiatsu, emphasizing its scientific principles and effects on muscle relaxation, circulation, and organ function.

In a Shiatsu session, practitioners use fingers, palms, and elbows to apply pressure to specific points along the meridians. These movements are deliberate and applied with rhythmic intensity to stimulate the body's natural healing response. Stretches and rotations are incorporated to support the flow of Qi (energy) and blood, balancing internal systems and promoting relaxation.

Today, Shiatsu has a broad, integrative approach. Practitioners may adapt techniques depending on the individual's needs, addressing physical, mental, and emotional aspects of health. As a natural therapy, Shiatsu does not use oils or lotions and is often performed with the recipient fully clothed, following the Japanese tradition of respecting personal space and privacy while focusing purely on energy manipulation.

Key Benefits For Stress Relief, Muscle Recovery, And Energy Balance

Shiatsu provides multiple benefits, particularly for stress relief, muscle relaxation, and energy balance. Targeting tension points along the body's meridians helps reduce stress, alleviate headaches, and ease muscle tightness. During the session, the practitioner uses steady, controlled pressure on specific areas, encouraging the release of endorphins and reducing cortisol levels, which contribute to an overall sense of calm.

For muscle recovery, Shiatsu is ideal because it targets both surface and deep muscle layers, encouraging blood circulation and lymph flow. Techniques like pressing, holding, and kneading are designed to promote recovery by clearing lactic acid build-up and releasing muscle tension. This makes Shiatsu particularly helpful for athletes or those recovering from physical strain.

Energy balance is another core benefit, as Shiatsu directly addresses the body's Qi. By working on meridian points, Shiatsu aims to restore balance, revitalize areas of low energy, and calm overactive zones. This energy harmonization supports a sense of physical vitality, emotional stability, and mental clarity, making Shiatsu a powerful practice for ongoing health and wellness.

Basic Principles Of Energy Flow And Meridian Lines

The meridian lines in Shiatsu are pathways through which Qi, or life energy, flows, connecting organs, muscles, and other body parts. Each meridian corresponds to a specific organ, such as the heart, liver, or lungs, and runs across various points in the body. When energy flows smoothly along these meridians, the body stays balanced; however, blockages in these pathways can lead to discomfort or illness.

In practice, Shiatsu addresses energy flow by pressing specific points along these meridians. For example, pressure on the stomach meridian, located on the front of the body, may relieve indigestion or abdominal discomfort.

Practitioners use a series of thumb, finger, or palm pressure, gradually moving along the meridian lines with a gentle, flowing rhythm to encourage the release of blockages.

Awareness of meridian lines is important for both the practitioner and receiver. Practitioners are trained to sense disruptions in energy flow, while recipients can support the process by staying relaxed and focused on their breathing. The synergy of breathing, pressure, and body awareness helps open up blocked meridians, restoring balance and promoting holistic healing.

Understanding The Body's Pressure Points

Pressure points, or Tsubo, are the locations along meridian lines where energy gathers and can be accessed for healing. Each point has a unique effect on the body and is chosen based on the individual's needs. For instance, pressing specific points on the back of the neck may help relieve tension headaches, while points along the lower back can alleviate sciatic pain.

To apply Shiatsu pressure effectively, practitioners use the thumb or finger to press directly into the Tsubo for a few seconds, gradually increasing and releasing pressure. The pressure should feel firm but comfortable, never painful. Holding pressure on a point can trigger a reflex that releases muscle tightness and enhances blood flow, while rhythmic pressing helps to re-energize fatigued areas.

Beginners can start by practicing on simple pressure points such as those on the hands and feet. These areas are accessible and offer relief for general tension and fatigue. For example, pressing on the "Hegu" point between the thumb and index finger can help relieve headaches and promote relaxation, making it an ideal starting point for self-care Shiatsu practice.

Essential Safety Tips And Contraindications

Shiatsu is generally safe, but it's essential to follow certain precautions to avoid injury or discomfort. Practitioners should always communicate with recipients to ensure that the pressure is comfortable. Too much pressure can cause soreness or bruising, particularly if someone has sensitive skin or underlying health issues. Avoid using strong pressure on sensitive areas like the spine or over-inflamed joints.

Contraindications include conditions such as fractures, recent surgery, and infections.

Pregnant individuals should also seek advice before receiving Shiatsu, as certain points can stimulate uterine contractions. People with osteoporosis, blood clotting disorders, or high blood pressure should consult a healthcare provider before starting Shiatsu, as some techniques may not be suitable.

For beginners practicing on themselves or others, starting gently and avoiding pressure on areas of known injury or sensitivity is wise. Regular practice helps develop sensitivity to the body's needs and energy flow, making it easier to adapt Shiatsu to individual circumstances.

CHAPTER TWO

Preparing For A Shiatsu Session

Setting Up A Relaxing And Comfortable Space

To create an optimal environment for Shiatsu, begin by finding a quiet, comfortable room where distractions and noise are minimal. Dim the lights slightly, and consider using candles or a diffuser with essential oils like lavender to enhance relaxation.

Ensure that the room temperature is comfortably warm, as the body tends to cool down during relaxation. Arrange the space so you and the recipient can move freely, with enough room to apply the various techniques without obstruction.

Choosing The Right Tools And Mats

The choice of mats is essential in Shiatsu to provide adequate support and comfort for the recipient. Traditional Shiatsu is often practiced on a futon-style mat placed on the floor, which allows both comfort and flexibility. Mats should be firm enough to support pressure without causing discomfort. A good Shiatsu mat should also be easily washable, as hygiene is crucial. Additionally, have a small pillow for head or knee support if the recipient needs extra comfort. Soft towels can also be handy to place under sensitive areas for additional support.

Grounding Techniques For The Practitioner

Before starting, grounding techniques help the practitioner focus, bringing a calm, centered state to the session. Take a few moments to stand with your feet hip-width apart, relax your shoulders, and let your arms hang naturally.

Breathe deeply, feeling your connection to the ground and visualizing a sense of stability through your legs and feet. Grounding enhances your balance and focus, enabling you to apply consistent, gentle pressure. Practitioners can also try focusing on their heartbeat to promote a calm, even rhythm to their movements throughout the session.

Hygiene And Basic Self-Care Practices Before Starting

Maintaining good hygiene is essential to both the practitioner's and the recipient's comfort.

Wash your hands thoroughly with warm water and soap before each session and ensure your nails are trimmed and clean to avoid accidental scratches.

Practitioners should also dress in loose, comfortable clothing that allows freedom of movement and prevents any restrictive feeling during body maneuvers. It's also recommended to stay hydrated and avoid strong perfumes, as some recipients may have sensitivities to smells.

How To Prepare The Recipient Physically And Mentally

To prepare the recipient, have them change into loose, comfortable clothing that allows movement and does not restrict circulation.

Invite them to take a few deep breaths to settle into the space and let go of any mental stress.

Explain briefly what they can expect during the session, such as gentle stretches and rhythmic pressure applied to various points on the body. This helps ease any anxiety and builds trust, allowing the recipient to fully relax and benefit from the Shiatsu techniques you'll be applying.

CHAPTER THREE

Basic Shiatsu Techniques For Beginners

Shiatsu, a Japanese technique that uses finger pressure to stimulate energy points, helps improve overall well-being and restore balance to the body. For beginners, the core principles focus on simplicity and precision. Start by locating specific acupoints, like those along the back, neck, and shoulders. Apply gentle, sustained pressure using your thumbs or fingers, easing into each press. For a comfortable experience, ensure your hands are warm and relaxed, as this helps facilitate a natural flow of energy.

Positioning is vital in Shiatsu. Sit or kneel comfortably next to the recipient, allowing you to access their body without straining. Keep your elbows slightly bent, as rigidity in the joints disrupts energy flow. For added balance, shift your weight subtly as you press, avoiding forceful jabs. Rhythmically use both hands, alternating between soft and moderate pressure. This steady, unhurried pace allows the body to respond positively, encouraging a deep sense of relaxation.

Practice patience and mindfulness. Begin with short sessions, focusing on mastering each point without rushing. The emphasis should always be on consistency and gentleness rather than intensity. As you get more comfortable with these basic techniques, increase the duration gradually, refining your sensitivity to the body's natural energy flows.

Remember that Shiatsu is as much about mental clarity as it is physical technique, so remain focused and receptive to the body's subtle feedback.

Introduction To Finger Pressure And Body-Weight Techniques

Finger pressure is the cornerstone of Shiatsu, aiming to stimulate vital energy points with steady, controlled movements. Position the tip of your thumb on a chosen point, applying gentle pressure for a few seconds, then release slowly. Avoid pressing too hard; Shiatsu focuses on harmonizing rather than forcing energy. To enhance the effect, use your entire thumb or finger pad to increase surface contact, ensuring each touch feels calming and grounding.

Body-weight techniques are key to generating consistent pressure without muscle strain. Instead of using just the strength in your arms, lean in gently with your body weight, shifting it onto the area. This allows your touch to feel firm but not overwhelming, giving the receiver a sense of support and relaxation. This method works particularly well along larger muscle groups like the back or thighs, where a broader touch helps ease tension.

To master body-weight techniques, maintain a straight posture and breathe deeply as you press. This helps channel your weight evenly, keeping the experience comfortable for both the giver and receiver. It's essential to keep your movements fluid and intentional, letting your weight carry naturally rather than pushing or forcing pressure. This technique allows even novice practitioners to offer a steady and therapeutic touch.

How To Apply Sustained Pressure On Energy Points

Sustained pressure is at the heart of Shiatsu's therapeutic effects, helping to release blocked energy and soothe tight muscles. To apply this effectively, choose a specific acupoint, like those along the spine or the base of the neck, and place the tip of your thumb or finger firmly on the spot. Gradually increase pressure over a few seconds until you feel resistance, holding for around 5-10 seconds without shifting.

While maintaining pressure, ensure your breathing remains steady and even, as this encourages the body to relax deeply. Use your body weight to sustain the pressure, keeping your arms relaxed. As you hold, be aware of subtle feedback from the body; if you feel a shift in muscle tension, it's a sign that the body is responding, and you may release gradually. Avoid sudden changes in pressure, as consistency is crucial to successful Shiatsu.

Once you release the hold, pause briefly to let the energy adjust. If needed, you can repeat the process, gradually moving along other nearby points. This technique is powerful when applied consistently, making it a valuable method for targeting persistent areas of tension. By practicing sustained pressure thoughtfully, you can deliver a deeply calming

Shiatsu experience that encourages energy to flow more freely.

Using Palms, Thumbs, And Elbows Effectively

Each body part used in Shiatsu serves a unique purpose. Palms are excellent for broader areas like the back and thighs, providing a comforting and steady touch. Place both palms gently on the target area and press down evenly with your body weight, holding for a few moments before releasing. This technique delivers a warming effect and can help relieve tension in large muscle groups.

Thumbs allow for more focused work on specific points along the shoulders, neck, or arms.

To avoid fatigue, use the base of your thumb rather than the tip, applying steady, moderate pressure. Move slowly, using small circles to enhance blood flow. This precise approach is useful for targeting smaller muscles or areas needing detailed attention, especially around joints.

Elbows offer even deeper pressure and are ideal for sturdy muscles, like those along the lower back or hips. To avoid discomfort, make sure your elbow is padded by gently placing a soft cloth between your elbow and the skin. Rest the elbow at a 45-degree angle on the point, leaning in gently. This method allows a robust yet controlled force, helping release deep-seated tension effectively without overstressing your hands or thumbs.

Simple Stretching Techniques For Flexibility

Stretching in Shiatsu helps improve flexibility and release muscular tension, making it a valuable addition to the technique. Begin with gentle stretches for areas like the shoulders and neck, where tension often accumulates. For shoulder stretches, place one hand on the shoulder and use the other to support the arm. Carefully lift and rotate the arm in small circles, letting the movement ease tension naturally.

For the lower back, gently bend the recipient's knee and guide it towards their chest, supporting the movement with your hands. Avoid forcing the stretch; let gravity do the work to keep it comfortable and effective. This slow, controlled motion enhances flexibility and encourages circulation to the area, often bringing relief to tight hip and lower back muscles.

To stretch the legs, hold the foot with one hand and support the knee with the other, slowly lifting the leg toward the chest. Move gradually, adjusting the stretch based on the recipient's comfort level. This technique aids in loosening muscles along the back of the legs, improving the range of motion. Shiatsu stretching should always be gentle, with each motion serving as a preparation for deeper, more sustained pressure work.

Flowing From One Area To Another For Smooth Energy Transitions

Smooth transitions between areas in Shiatsu enhance the flow of energy, making the treatment feel seamless and harmonious. Start with the shoulders, pressing gently with your thumbs, and gradually move down to the lower back. Instead of lifting your hands abruptly, slide them naturally, maintaining a light touch to keep the energy connected. This flow helps prevent interruptions in the body's energy fields.

As you move from one part to another, maintain rhythm and pace, giving each area sufficient time to relax. Transitioning can be as simple as shifting from shoulders to arms in one fluid motion. After finishing one area, let your hands lightly "glide" to the next, keeping contact at all times. These smooth movements help the receiver feel grounded, enhancing the overall relaxation experience.

Ensure that each transition is mindful and intentional, bringing calm and balance to each part of the body. This steady flow creates a cohesive experience, which is especially valuable in Shiatsu, where maintaining an uninterrupted energy line is key to restoring balance. Flowing transitions help unify the session, allowing both the giver and receiver to feel centered and fully immersed in the healing process.

CHAPTER FOUR

Shiatsu For Stress Reduction

Shiatsu can be highly effective for stress relief, involving gentle pressure applied through the hands, palms, and thumbs to reduce tension. Begin by taking a seated position with feet flat on the ground or lying on a comfortable surface. Focus on deep, slow breathing to help relax the body and prepare it for the technique.

Use your thumbs to press lightly at the base of the skull where the neck meets the head—this is known as the suboccipital area. Maintain gentle, sustained pressure for about five seconds, releasing and repeating a few times. This approach relaxes the neck and shoulders, releasing tension that accumulates due to stress.

Next, apply light to moderate pressure along the trapezius muscles, located between the neck and shoulder. Using your thumbs or fingertips, press and hold for several seconds at different points along the muscle, moving from the base of the neck out toward the shoulder. This helps alleviate tightness and reduce stress stored in the shoulder area. Pay attention to your breathing, synchronizing each press with a slow inhale and exhale. To deepen relaxation, apply this technique to both shoulders, maintaining a comfortable, even pressure.

Finish by gently massaging the base of the spine with your thumbs or knuckles. The lower back often holds residual tension from prolonged stress, so place your thumbs along the sacrum, the bony area at the base of the spine, and apply light circular motions. This movement helps release the body's energy flow and promotes a sense of calm. Regular practice of these simple techniques can effectively reduce stress and enhance well-being.

Key Pressure Points For Calming The Nervous System

Key pressure points play a central role in calming the nervous system through shiatsu. One of the primary points is the "Yintang," located between the eyebrows. To activate this, gently place your thumb or index finger on this point and apply soft pressure, holding for about five to ten seconds while breathing deeply. This helps soothe the mind, alleviate headaches, and reduce anxiety. Make sure to maintain a slow, rhythmic breathing pattern as you press; this enhances relaxation.

Another essential pressure point is the "Hegu," located in the webbing between the thumb and index finger. Hold this area with gentle yet firm pressure for about five seconds, then release. This technique helps reduce mental stress and promotes the release of endorphins, the body's natural feel-good hormones.

Repeat on both hands, applying pressure in sync with deep breathing to increase relaxation. This can be done any time you need a quick calming effect, as it's simple and discreet.

The final key point is the "Anmian," located behind the ear at the base of the skull. Gently press with your fingertips on this point for about ten seconds, then release. This area is highly effective for promoting restful sleep and easing anxiety. Press gently, moving in small circles to release tension around the area. Regularly applying pressure on these points can help regulate your nervous system, encouraging an overall calm state.

Techniques For Relieving Tension In Shoulders And Neck

To relieve tension in the shoulders, start by using your thumbs to apply steady pressure along the trapezius muscle at the top of the shoulder. Move in small circular motions from the base of the neck toward the shoulder joint, applying moderate pressure.

This helps release built-up tension in the muscles that often become strained due to stress and poor posture. Be mindful of your breathing, exhaling deeply with each press to aid muscle relaxation.

Next, move to the neck area. Use your fingertips to gently press along the sides of the neck from just below the skull toward the base of the neck. Apply soft pressure for three to five seconds at each point, moving slowly down the neck.

This technique targets the muscles that carry tension from long hours of sitting or stress and can promote blood flow and relaxation. Avoid pressing directly on the spine and instead work along the muscle lines for optimal comfort.

To finish, apply light tapping along the shoulder and neck area with relaxed fists. This tapping action helps improve circulation and relieve any remaining tightness in the upper body.

Work gently but rhythmically, ensuring you don't over-tap or apply too much force. With consistent practice, these techniques help alleviate chronic shoulder and neck tension, bringing lasting relief and ease to these common areas of discomfort.

Gentle Pressure Applications For Relaxation

For gentle shiatsu pressure application, start with the forearms and wrists. Place one hand on the opposite forearm, using your thumb to press gently but steadily along the inner side of the arm, moving toward the wrist. This area often holds tension, so keep your grip light, maintaining each press for about three seconds before moving to the next spot. This encourages circulation and promotes a sense of relaxation in the arms and hands.

Continue with gentle pressure on the back, particularly along the spine. Place your palms on either side of the spine at the upper back, using the heel of your hand to apply light pressure.

Move slowly down the spine, pressing gently at each point along the back. Avoid pressing directly on the spine itself, instead focusing on the muscles on either side. This technique soothes the central nervous system, reducing stress and promoting relaxation.

To conclude, apply gentle circular motions to the temples. Place your fingertips on your temples and move them in small, soft circles, which can relieve headaches and help you unwind.

Apply light pressure, and take slow breaths as you perform the motions. This gentle touch approach is ideal for beginners looking to introduce relaxation techniques into their routine, as it eases both the mind and body.

Step-By-Step Sequences For Stress Relief

Begin your stress-relief shiatsu sequence with deep breathing exercises, inhaling through the nose and exhaling through the mouth. Place your thumbs on the base of the skull and press gently, holding for a few seconds.

Release and move down the neck, applying light pressure at various points.

This sequence helps relax the upper body and soothes the nervous system.

Next, focus on the shoulders. With fingertips or thumbs, apply pressure along the shoulders, from the neck to the shoulder joint, moving in small circles. Hold each point for three seconds before moving to the next, ensuring a steady rhythm.

Pay attention to your breathing, inhaling as you press and exhaling as you release. This shoulder work relieves physical stress and enhances blood flow, leaving you feeling lighter.

Finish with a gentle hand massage, applying pressure along the fingers and palms. Start at the base of each finger, pressing lightly as you move up to the tip. Then, press along the palm in small circles, focusing on any tense areas.

End by gently massaging the wrists, as this supports relaxation and stress relief for the entire body. Practicing this step-by-step sequence regularly can become an effective part of managing everyday stress.

Tips For Creating A Soothing Environment

Creating a calm setting is essential for effective shiatsu practice. Start by choosing a quiet, comfortable room with minimal distractions.

Dim the lights or use a soft, warm light source to create a relaxing atmosphere, as bright lighting can be overly stimulating. You may also consider using a soft mat or cushion to make seated or lying positions more comfortable, as this allows for full-body relaxation during the session. Incorporate soothing sounds or gentle music that promotes relaxation. Nature sounds like ocean waves or birdsong can help center the mind and reduce stress.

Additionally, essential oils like lavender or chamomile can enhance the calming effects. Diffuse a few drops or apply a small amount on your wrists to promote a grounding atmosphere, helping you focus on the shiatsu practice with ease.

Lastly, wear loose, comfortable clothing that allows free movement and proper circulation. Avoid tight or restrictive outfits, as comfort is key to a successful shiatsu experience. Keep a blanket or shawl nearby to keep warm, especially in cooler environments.

By creating an inviting, tranquil space, you'll find it easier to fully immerse yourself in the process, making each shiatsu session more effective for stress relief.

CHAPTER FIVE

Shiatsu For Muscle Recovery

Identifying Muscle Pain And Tension Areas

To begin a shiatsu session focused on muscle recovery, identifying areas of pain or tension is crucial. Start by gently pressing different muscle groups, noting any areas of tightness, soreness, or sensitivity. Pay particular attention to common trouble spots like the shoulders, neck, lower back, thighs, and calves, which often carry the most tension. Use your thumbs and fingers to explore these muscles, applying gentle pressure and moving slowly to assess where relief may be needed most.

Once you've identified areas of tension, consider the type of discomfort: is it a dull ache, sharp pain, or stiffness? Different sensations can indicate varying levels of muscle strain or injury, and recognizing this helps in selecting the most effective pressure techniques. For deeper, aching pains, you may want to use slower, firmer pressure, while for sharper pain, a gentler approach can prevent aggravation. This preliminary assessment helps to personalize the treatment and better target specific needs.

Incorporate some mindful breathing as you explore these areas, which can help both the practitioner and recipient relax and become more aware of bodily sensations. During this process, encourage the person receiving shiatsu to communicate openly about any discomfort or relief felt, helping guide the process for optimal muscle recovery.

Techniques For Relieving Soreness And Enhancing Circulation

Relieving muscle soreness with shiatsu involves applying sustained pressure along tense areas to help release the tightness. Start by using your thumbs to press gently into the muscle, gradually increasing pressure as tolerated. Work in a slow, circular motion around the muscle, avoiding any direct pressure on bones or joints. This technique boosts blood circulation, helping muscles relax and encouraging the body's natural healing process.

An effective shiatsu approach is the "press-and-hold" method. Apply pressure to a specific point on the muscle for 5-10 seconds, then release slowly. This technique is especially useful in areas like the shoulders and back, where tension tends to build up. Once pressure is released, you may notice the muscle feels warmer and looser, which indicates increased blood flow to the area.

You can also try the "kneading" technique, where you gently grasp and lift the muscle tissue with your fingers, simulating a gentle massage. This helps to reduce muscle stiffness, allowing improved circulation to areas previously starved of oxygen. Always follow up with a soft, gliding motion to help transition between areas smoothly, maintaining relaxation and avoiding any abrupt changes in pressure.

Using Pressure Points To Support Muscle Repair

Shiatsu focuses heavily on the use of pressure points, called "tsubo," which are specific areas along the body that can help promote muscle healing when stimulated. Begin by applying gentle pressure to points known for muscle relief, such as Gallbladder 21 (GB21) at the shoulder's top, often effective for neck and shoulder tension. Use your thumb to apply steady pressure for 5-7 seconds, then release and repeat several times.

Another essential point for muscle recovery is Bladder 23 (BL23), located on either side of the lower back. To stimulate this area, use your palms or thumbs to apply firm pressure for 10 seconds, then release. This technique helps reduce lower back tension and supports the kidneys, which play a role in the body's healing processes.

For leg and calf pain, try the Stomach 36 (ST36) point, which lies four fingers below the kneecap. Press firmly with your thumb and hold for a few seconds, feeling the muscle relax. Incorporating these specific points during a shiatsu session promotes natural muscle recovery and reduces soreness by enhancing circulation and the body's self-healing abilities.

Step-By-Step Recovery Session Examples

To start a muscle recovery session, position the recipient comfortably on a mat or chair. Begin by warming up the muscles with gentle pressure across the entire body, focusing initially on large muscle groups like the back and legs. Use your palms to apply gentle pressure along the spine and thighs, gradually increasing it to create a sense of relaxation and openness in the muscles.

Move on to the targeted pressure points for muscle relief, such as GB21 and BL23, using a mix of pressing and holding techniques as well as light kneading. Work slowly and mindfully, focusing on areas previously identified as tense or sore, maintaining consistent pressure for optimal muscle relaxation and blood flow. Allow the recipient to take deep breaths, encouraging further relaxation with each exhale.

Finish the session with a calming full-body sweep using your palms to gently glide over the body, easing any lingering tension and promoting a balanced feeling. This step helps integrate the benefits of the shiatsu session, leaving the recipient feeling refreshed and aiding in faster recovery.

Self-Shiatsu Techniques For Muscle Recovery

Self-shiatsu for muscle recovery can be easily done on commonly strained areas like the shoulders, neck, and legs.

Start by sitting comfortably, and place your fingers or thumbs on your shoulders, pressing gently along the muscles from the neck to the shoulder tip. Apply moderate pressure and hold for a few seconds, releasing gradually before moving to the next spot.

For sore legs, use both thumbs to apply pressure along the calf and thigh muscles. Work upwards from the ankle to the knee, then from the knee to the thigh. Use a pressing and releasing motion as you work, spending extra time on areas that feel particularly tight. Repeat this process on each leg, aiming for a balanced application of pressure on both sides of the body.

To release neck tension, place your thumbs on the base of your skull and apply gentle circular pressure, moving down toward the shoulders. This is effective for people who sit at desks or carry heavy loads. Practicing self-shiatsu on these areas after a workout or long day helps maintain muscle health, reduces soreness, and supports the body's recovery process.

CHAPTER SIX

Shiatsu For Energy Balancing

Shiatsu is a therapeutic technique originating from Japan that uses finger pressure on specific areas of the body to harmonize the flow of energy, known as Ki or Qi. Practitioners believe energy blockages or imbalances lead to fatigue and stress.

Shiatsu helps restore balance by stimulating acupressure points along the body's energy channels, known as meridians, to encourage a free and steady energy flow. You can perform these techniques on yourself or a partner to improve vitality and promote well-being.

Understanding The Body's Energy Meridians

The meridians are invisible channels through which life energy flows, corresponding to various organs like the heart, lungs, and stomach. In Shiatsu, twelve major meridians run symmetrically along both sides of the body.

For example, the stomach meridian runs from under the eye down the chest to the feet, while the bladder meridian extends along the back. Learning these meridian paths is crucial since blockages in one area may affect distant parts of the body. Recognizing these energy highways allows you to target the right pressure points for better energy flow.

Techniques For Balancing Energy Flow And Boosting Vitality

Use the palms, thumbs, or knuckles to apply steady pressure along the meridians, holding each point for 5-7 seconds before releasing. For example, press gently into the space between your thumb and index finger (the Large Intestine 4 point) to relieve fatigue.

The pressure should be firm but not painful, and you can enhance its effect by breathing deeply through your nose.

For a quick energy boost, rub your hands together briskly and place them on the kidneys (lower back), using circular movements to stimulate warmth and flow.

Key Points Along The Meridians For Energy Boost

Several points can increase energy when stimulated. One essential point is the "Kidney 1" (Yongquan), located on the sole, which grounds the body's energy. The "Stomach 36" point (Zusanli), located four fingers below the kneecap and one finger width to the outside, is known as the energy-enhancing point. When applying pressure to these areas, use your thumb in a circular motion for about 30 seconds. Activating these key points not only relieves fatigue but also improves circulation, digestion, and mental clarity.

Simple Routines For Morning Energy Enhancement

Start your morning with a 5-minute Shiatsu routine to wake up your energy.

Begin by rubbing your palms together to generate heat and place them over your eyes. Next, gently tap along your arms, starting from the shoulders down to your fingertips, stimulating the lung meridian. Massage the kidney area on your lower back with circular motions to activate energy flow, followed by light tapping along the legs to energize your body. Finish by pressing the Stomach 36 point for 15-30 seconds on each leg to boost stamina.

End-Of-Day Routines For Energy Rebalancing

At the end of the day, a calming Shiatsu routine helps restore balance and prepare for sleep. Start by sitting comfortably and using your thumbs to press gently along your eyebrows and temples, releasing built-up tension. Massage the soles of your feet, focusing on the Kidney 1 point, to relax the mind and ground your energy. Use both hands to apply gentle pressure along the bladder meridian on your lower back, releasing stiffness from sitting or standing. Finish with deep, mindful breathing while pressing the Heart 7 point (located at the wrist crease) to calm your nervous system and promote restful sleep.

CHAPTER SEVEN

Special Techniques For Common Ailments

Shiatsu techniques are ideal for addressing everyday ailments, focusing on pressure points to relieve discomfort and promote energy flow. For example, to address tight muscles, use your thumbs or palms to apply firm but gentle pressure to the affected area. Hold the pressure for a few seconds, then release, gradually increasing as the muscles begin to relax. This process helps to release tension and improve circulation, which is beneficial for soreness.

Another common technique involves using the knuckles to massage more rigid areas, such as the shoulder blades.

Make a fist, then use the knuckles to apply pressure to the shoulder, moving in circular motions. This can alleviate tension from prolonged sitting or poor posture. Focus on even, rhythmic pressure to achieve the best results and avoid strain.

To finish, light tapping with the edges of the hands, known as percussion, can be effective. Gently tap along the spine or tense muscles in the neck, helping to stimulate blood flow and release stress from these areas.

These techniques, used individually or combined, offer targeted relief and can be adapted to a range of common issues, allowing for daily practice.

Techniques For Headaches And Sinus Relief

For headaches, Shiatsu focuses on pressure points in the head, neck, and face. Begin by using your thumbs to press gently at the temples, moving in circular motions for about 10–15 seconds. Next, work from the center of the forehead, above the eyebrows, and move outward toward the temples. This promotes circulation and helps alleviate tension that often builds in these areas.

To relieve sinus discomfort, press gently on the points beside the nostrils and move upward along the sides of the nose toward the cheekbones. Hold these points for a few seconds, then release and repeat. This can reduce sinus pressure and open nasal passages.

Massaging around the eyes in circular motions may also improve sinus drainage, relieving pressure and tension.

Finally, work down the back of the head and neck by applying thumb pressure along the base of the skull. This relieves tension in the neck, which is often connected to headaches. Remember to breathe deeply throughout and keep your movements slow to encourage relaxation and improve blood flow in these areas.

Relieving Lower Back Pain And Tension
For lower back pain, start by using the palms of your hands to press along the lower spine and sacrum. Applying gentle but firm pressure along the spine's muscles can help to release tension in the lower back.

Move in a slow, circular motion with the heel of your hand, focusing on relaxing the muscles near the spine.

You can also use your thumbs to apply pressure to specific points along the lower back, such as the dimples just above the hips (known as the sacroiliac points). Press these points firmly, hold for several seconds, and release. This can help ease stiffness and reduce tension in the muscles around the hips and lower back, which are often strained from sitting or lifting.

Another effective technique is to use knuckles to massage the muscles on either side of the spine. Starting at the base of the spine, work your way upward to just below the ribcage, applying firm but comfortable pressure.

This movement stimulates blood flow and releases tension in the lower back muscles, making it particularly helpful for people with chronic back pain.

Shiatsu For Digestive Issues And Abdominal Discomfort

Shiatsu for digestive issues involves focusing on the abdomen and lower back to improve digestion. Begin by applying gentle pressure in circular motions around the navel. Start with light pressure and gradually increase as the abdomen relaxes. This massage helps stimulate the intestines and relieve constipation or bloating.

Next, use your fingertips to press along the stomach area in a clockwise motion. This direction follows the natural path of digestion and can be soothing for cramping or gas pain. Hold each point for a few seconds before moving to the next, focusing on areas that feel tense or uncomfortable.

Lastly, apply gentle pressure along the sides of the lower abdomen. Pressing these points can help alleviate discomfort related to indigestion and encourage a sense of calm. Try incorporating deep breathing as you work on these points, as it promotes relaxation and helps reduce stress, which can also aid in digestive health.

Techniques For Improving Sleep Quality
Shiatsu can be a valuable tool for improving sleep by focusing on points that encourage relaxation and release physical tension. Start with gentle pressure on the top of the head

using your fingertips. Apply slight circular motions for a few minutes, which can calm the mind and relieve stress, making it easier to wind down before sleep.

Move to the center of the chest, applying light pressure with your fingertips in small, clockwise circles. This area, near the heart center, can promote a sense of calm and relaxation. Slow, rhythmic breathing while massaging this point encourages a calm state, helping reduce anxiety or restlessness.

Lastly, massage the soles of the feet using your thumbs in slow circular motions. Start at the base of the toes and work down to the heel. Applying pressure to the arches and outer edges is especially helpful for grounding the body. Practicing this nightly can make a noticeable difference in sleep quality over time.

Alleviating Fatigue With Targeted Points

To relieve fatigue, focus on points that enhance energy flow and reduce physical tension. Begin by using your thumbs to press at the center of the palms. Hold each pressure point for a few seconds, then release. This technique is believed to stimulate energy flow and refresh the body, making it a great morning routine.

Next, work on the point between the thumb and index finger. Press and hold for several seconds on each hand. This point is linked to relieving tension and boosting alertness, helping to reduce feelings of fatigue or mental fog. It's effective during mid-day slumps when you need a quick energy boost.

Finally, use your thumbs to massage along the back of the calves, especially around the Achilles tendon. This area is linked to circulation and can help refresh tired legs. By massaging these points, you can reinvigorate your energy levels, making it a practical way to recharge and improve focus throughout the day.

CHAPTER EIGHT

Self-Shiatsu For Personal Wellness

Basic Techniques For Daily Self-Care

Self-shiatsu, or self-massage using shiatsu techniques, begins with gentle pressing and kneading movements along your body's meridians, or energy pathways. To start, use your thumbs or fingers to apply steady pressure on areas like the shoulders, neck, and lower back. Breathe deeply as you press, allowing each point to be held for 5-7 seconds before releasing. When pressing down on a point, apply just enough pressure to feel slight discomfort—never pain—as this activates energy flow.

For areas where pressing with your fingers might be challenging, try using a tennis ball or foam roller. Place the ball on the floor and gently lean into it with the part of your body that needs attention, like your upper back or glutes. This is particularly helpful for larger muscle areas. Moving gently back and forth over the ball can enhance circulation, release tension, and stimulate acupressure points.

Incorporate self-shiatsu into your day by dedicating a few minutes in the morning or before bed. It's a practice that aligns well with deep breathing exercises, helping you focus on your body and relax mentally. This consistent routine brings physical benefits and enhances body awareness, gradually building mindfulness that can be calming and restorative.

Key Pressure Points You Can Reach Yourself

Several accessible pressure points can be stimulated for various benefits, from relieving headaches to soothing tense muscles. One popular point is the "Third Eye," located between the eyebrows.

Using your middle finger, apply gentle pressure here for a minute, which can help alleviate stress and mental fatigue. Another key point is LI-4, between the thumb and index finger; pressing this spot can relieve headache tension and even reduce anxiety.

Another effective point is GB-20, at the base of the skull, where the neck meets the back of the head.

To stimulate GB-20, interlock your fingers and gently press your thumbs into the area on both sides of the neck's midline.

Hold the pressure for 10-15 seconds while taking slow, deep breaths, which can alleviate neck pain, tension, and eye strain from screen exposure.

For lower back tension, try pressing the B-23 and B-47 points, located roughly two finger-widths from each side of your spine at waist level.

While sitting, apply firm pressure using your thumbs and massage in a circular motion for around 10 seconds. These points help relieve lower back pain and ease tension, offering a way to release stress accumulated from long hours of sitting.

Techniques For Reducing Daily Stress And Fatigue

Shiatsu for stress relief focuses on slow, firm pressure applied to areas like the shoulders, neck, and lower back, where tension often accumulates.

To start, gently press into the "shoulder well" (GB-21) between the shoulder and neck, massaging with your fingertips. Press firmly but comfortably, and breathe deeply, as this technique relaxes tight shoulder muscles and stimulates blood flow.

The area around the temples and jaw is also beneficial for tension release. Using two fingers, apply light pressure in circular motions on your temples, then move down to the jawline, which can ease mental fatigue and stress. You can also gently press your palms against the sides of your head, holding for a few seconds, which can relax the mind and alleviate headaches from mental strain.

For energy and mood improvement, apply light tapping motions along the sides of your arms and legs. This technique, often called "percussive shiatsu," activates blood flow and can stimulate energy levels.

As you tap, take deep breaths and try to visualize tension leaving your body, which enhances the technique's benefits by grounding and calming you.

Morning And Evening Self-Routines

Start your morning with a quick self-shiatsu routine to boost energy. Begin by gently pressing the LI-4 point between your thumb and index finger on each hand for 10 seconds, releasing, then repeating. This can help wake up your system and release morning stiffness. Move to the area around your temples, using gentle circular motions to reduce grogginess. This entire routine can be completed in under 5 minutes and helps set a positive, energized tone for your day.

For an evening routine, try a calming sequence that targets the shoulders, neck, and lower back. Start with deep breaths to center yourself, then press down on the "heavenly pillar" points (B-10), located just below the base of the skull. Hold each point for a few seconds, which can relax neck tension and promote restful sleep. Next, gently press along your lower back, especially the B-23 points, which support kidney energy and help unwind physical tension.

To complete your nighttime shiatsu routine, lie down and place a tennis ball beneath each shoulder blade, moving slowly from side to side. This technique helps release deeper layers of muscle tension, allowing you to let go of the day's stresses and easing the body into a restful state. Finish by stretching out fully, and taking three deep breaths to settle into relaxation before sleep.

Precautions And Limitations Of Self-Shiatsu

While self-shiatsu is generally safe, it's essential to understand your body's limits and never apply too much pressure, especially in sensitive areas. Beginners should start with gentle techniques and increase intensity gradually, always avoiding any pressure that leads to sharp or intense pain. If you experience ongoing pain or discomfort, consult a healthcare professional to ensure it's safe to continue self-shiatsu.

Avoid using shiatsu on areas of the body where there is inflammation, bruising, or broken skin, as pressing these areas could worsen symptoms. Similarly, it's best to avoid shiatsu in specific health conditions, like recent surgeries or severe joint issues, without professional guidance. Pregnant individuals should exercise additional caution, as certain points can trigger contractions.

Finally, remember that shiatsu complements but does not replace medical care. Self-shiatsu can be beneficial for relaxation and stress management, but it is not a substitute for professional treatments if you have chronic conditions. Incorporate it as a supportive practice, respecting your body's needs and limitations, to enjoy the best results safely.

CHAPTER NINE

Common Concerns And FAQs

Shiatsu is a popular form of Japanese massages therapy that utilizes finger pressure on specific points of the body to promote relaxation and healing. One common concern is the intensity of pressure used during the treatment. Beginners should communicate openly with their practitioners about their comfort levels, as Shiatsu should not cause pain. Practitioners typically adjust their techniques based on the individual's needs, ensuring a balance between therapeutic pressure and relaxation.

Another frequent question revolves around the settings in which Shiatsu can be performed.

While it's often offered in spas or wellness centers, Shiatsu can also be practiced in more casual environments, such as at home or even at work. Learning basic techniques can empower individuals to perform simple Shiatsu on themselves or friends, enhancing relaxation and well-being without requiring a formal session.

Lastly, many people inquire about the qualifications of Shiatsu practitioners. It's essential to choose a certified professional with proper training in Shiatsu techniques and anatomy. This ensures that you receive safe and effective treatment tailored to your specific needs, whether you seek relief from stress, muscle tension, or other health issues.

How Often Can Shiatsu Be Practiced?

The frequency of Shiatsu sessions can vary based on individual health goals and needs. For beginners, it's often recommended to start with one session per week to establish a routine and gauge the body's response. This frequency allows for adequate time to integrate the benefits of each session while assessing how your body feels afterward. After a few weeks, you can adjust the frequency based on personal preferences and how your body responds to treatment.

For individuals seeking relief from specific conditions, such as chronic pain or stress, more frequent sessions—such as two to three times per week—may be beneficial initially. As symptoms improve, the frequency can be gradually reduced to bi-weekly or monthly sessions to maintain overall well-being. It's essential to listen to your body and consult with your practitioner for personalized recommendations.

In addition, some practitioners suggest integrating Shiatsu into your wellness routine alongside other self-care practices like yoga, meditation, or regular exercise. This holistic approach can enhance the overall benefits of Shiatsu, promoting balance and relaxation throughout your body and mind.

Is Shiatsu Safe For Children, Elderly, Or Pregnant People?

Shiatsu can be a safe and effective treatment for various demographics, including children, the elderly, and pregnant individuals.

For children, the pressure applied during Shiatsu is typically lighter and tailored to their smaller bodies. Parents should ensure that the practitioner is experienced in working with children, as they may require different techniques compared to adults. Regular Shiatsu sessions can support children's overall health, help with sleep issues, and enhance their immune systems.

For elderly individuals, Shiatsu can promote relaxation, improve circulation, and alleviate chronic pain. Practitioners often adjust techniques to accommodate age-related sensitivities and mobility issues. Elderly clients need to communicate their health conditions and any medications they are taking to ensure a safe and effective experience.

With proper care, Shiatsu can be an excellent complementary therapy for maintaining health in older adults.

Pregnant individuals can also benefit from Shiatsu, as it can help alleviate discomfort associated with pregnancy, such as back pain and swelling. However, it's crucial to consult with a healthcare provider before receiving Shiatsu during pregnancy, particularly in the first trimester. Many practitioners specialize in prenatal Shiatsu, adapting their techniques to ensure safety and comfort for both the mother and the baby.

What Should I Expect After A Shiatsu Session?

After a Shiatsu session, it's common to feel a sense of deep relaxation and a reduction in tension throughout the body. Many clients report a heightened awareness of their physical state, which can encourage mindfulness about their posture and movement. It's important to stay hydrated after the session, as this helps to flush out toxins released during the treatment and can enhance the overall benefits experienced.

Some individuals may experience mild soreness or fatigue after their first Shiatsu session, especially if they are not accustomed to bodywork. This is usually temporary and can be relieved by gentle stretching, hydration, and rest. If the discomfort persists or feels unusual, it's advisable to communicate with your practitioner to address any concerns and adjust future treatments accordingly.

Additionally, you may notice changes in your mood and energy levels after a session.

Shiatsu can help reduce stress and promote emotional well-being, allowing you to feel more balanced and centered. Keeping a journal of your feelings and physical sensations after each session can help track your progress and enhance the overall effectiveness of your Shiatsu experience.

How Does Shiatsu Compare To Other Massage Therapies?

Shiatsu is distinct from other massage therapies due to its focus on acupressure points and the concept of energy flow, or "Qi." Unlike Swedish or deep tissue massages, which primarily target muscles and tension, Shiatsu aims to balance energy within the body by applying pressure to specific meridian points. This approach can lead to more holistic benefits, addressing not only physical discomfort but also emotional and energetic imbalances.

Another key difference is that Shiatsu is typically performed on a futon or mat on the floor, rather than on a massage table. This positioning allows practitioners to use their body weight to apply pressure effectively and facilitates a greater range of motion for stretching and manipulation.

As a result, Shiatsu can feel more dynamic and comprehensive compared to traditional table massages, which often focus on specific muscle groups.

While both Shiatsu and other massage therapies offer relaxation and stress relief, the emphasis on energy flow and meridian work sets Shiatsu apart.

Those seeking a deeper understanding of their body's energy dynamics and looking for an integrative approach to wellness may find Shiatsu particularly beneficial as part of their holistic health journey.

Tips For Handling Soreness Or Light Discomfort

Experiencing mild soreness or discomfort after a Shiatsu session is common, especially for beginners. To manage this, it's essential to listen to your body and give yourself time to rest.

Gentle stretching can help alleviate tightness and increase blood flow to sore areas. Simple stretches like neck rolls, shoulder shrugs, and hamstring stretches can be effective in easing discomfort and promoting relaxation.

Hydration plays a crucial role in the recovery after Shiatsu. Drinking plenty of water helps flush out toxins released during the session, reducing the likelihood of lingering soreness. Herbal teas, particularly those known for their anti-inflammatory properties, like ginger or chamomile, can also support recovery and enhance overall relaxation.

If soreness persists or feels more intense than expected, consider applying heat or cold packs to the affected areas.

A warm compress can soothe muscle tension, while a cold pack can reduce inflammation. Always communicate with your Shiatsu practitioner about any discomfort you experience, as they can adjust future sessions to better meet your needs and enhance your overall comfort and healing process.

CHAPTER TEN

Shiatsu As A Journey – Developing Your Skills

Shiatsu is an evolving practice that requires time and dedication to master. As you progress, you'll learn to develop a deeper connection with both your body and the person you're working on. Start by focusing on the basics: proper posture, correct hand placement, and sensitivity to your partner's energy. Practicing regularly and applying techniques gently will help build a foundation for effective Shiatsu.

To advance your skills, focus on your breathing and the flow of energy (Qi) throughout your practice.

Allow each movement to be mindful, using your palms, thumbs, and fingers to apply pressure with precision. By tuning into the energy lines (meridians) and listening to your partner's body, you can deliver targeted relief. Learning new techniques, such as different forms of pressure or stretching, will enrich your practice.

Reflect on each session and note the areas where you can improve. Keep practicing on different people to gain insight into how different body types react to Shiatsu. This will broaden your understanding of the body's energy systems and develop your confidence as you see positive changes in your partners over time.

How To Continue Learning And Growing In Shiatsu

Shiatsu, like any therapeutic art, demands continuous learning. After mastering the basics, deepen your knowledge through workshops, online courses, or mentorships with experienced practitioners. It is important to stay open to learning about different styles and techniques, such as Namikoshi or Zen Shiatsu, to broaden your approach and understanding.

Attending live workshops allows for hands-on experience, which is crucial to improving your tactile sensitivity. As you practice, focus on refining your technique and listening to feedback from both teachers and clients. Remember to study anatomy and physiology, as understanding the body's structure will enhance your ability to locate meridians and key pressure points.

Reading books or joining Shiatsu groups will introduce you to new perspectives and methodologies. It's important to stay curious and adaptable, experimenting with different techniques until you find what works best for you and the people you work with. Continued growth in Shiatsu happens through consistent practice, learning, and reflection.

Tips For Building Confidence And Intuition

Building confidence in Shiatsu comes from repetition, feedback, and trusting your instincts. Begin by practicing with family or friends and be open to their input about how your touch feels. This will help you adjust your pressure and technique based on the feedback you receive, building trust in your skills over time.

Developing intuition is key to becoming a great Shiatsu practitioner. Focus on sensing the subtle energy shifts in the body. Close your eyes during sessions to heighten your sense of touch and allow your hands to "listen" to the body's needs. Trust your instincts about where to apply pressure and how deeply to go, while always being mindful of your client's comfort.

Keep practicing mindfulness and meditation to tune into your inner awareness. As you relax and trust your process, your confidence will naturally grow. Intuition becomes more reliable as you gain more experience, so don't rush the process—let it develop as you continue practicing.

Common Mistakes To Avoid In Practice

One common mistake beginners make in Shiatsu is applying too much pressure too soon. Shiatsu is about creating balance, so start with gentle pressure and gradually increase intensity based on your partner's reactions. Always communicate and ensure the person receiving the treatment feels comfortable and not in pain.

Another mistake is neglecting your own posture. Good posture is crucial for delivering effective Shiatsu without straining your own body. Always check your alignment, ensuring that you are applying pressure using your body weight, rather than muscle strength alone. This ensures both you and your partner benefit from the session.

Lastly, avoid rushing the process. Shiatsu is not about speed but rather about mindful and deliberate pressure. Take your time to feel each area of the body, observe the energy flow, and address any areas of tension. Moving too quickly reduces the effectiveness of the treatment and may lead to missed areas in need of attention.

Practicing Different Body Types

Different body types respond to Shiatsu in unique ways, so it's important to adapt your techniques based on the person you are working with. For larger or muscular individuals, you may need to apply deeper pressure to reach the muscles and meridians.

Use your elbows or knees in addition to your hands to provide the necessary force without straining yourself.

For smaller or more delicate body types, lighter pressure is often more effective. Focus on gentler techniques and be mindful of fragile areas, such as joints and bones. Using your palms and fingers to apply broad, even pressure can prevent discomfort while still offering therapeutic benefits.

When working with children or elderly individuals, adjust your techniques to be even more sensitive and gentle. The key to working with all body types is listening to the body's response and adapting your pressure accordingly. With experience, you'll learn how to modify your practice based on the needs of each individual.

Connecting With The Shiatsu Community And Resources For Further Learning

To grow in your Shiatsu practice, connecting with the broader Shiatsu community is essential. Join local Shiatsu groups or online forums where practitioners share their experiences and advice. These communities can offer valuable feedback, help troubleshoot challenges, and keep you updated on new techniques or approaches.

Participating in workshops, seminars, and certification courses also provides opportunities to network with fellow practitioners.

Many associations offer continuing education courses that deepen your understanding and skillset. You'll benefit from the shared wisdom of both experienced professionals and peers at your level.

Stay informed by reading books, watching instructional videos, and exploring Shiatsu blogs. Learning is a lifelong journey, and regularly engaging with new material will keep you motivated and inspired. Being part of a community ensures that you never stop improving, and you can always find support when needed.

Conclusion

In conclusion, this book presents a holistic, practical, and accessible approach to understanding and practicing the Japanese healing art of Shiatsu. Rooted in traditional Eastern medicine, Shiatsu focuses on restoring the body's energy flow (or "qi") through targeted pressure applied to specific points along the body's meridians. This method not only alleviates physical symptoms but also addresses underlying mental and emotional imbalances, promoting overall well-being.

One of this guide's key strengths is its comprehensive breakdown of various Shiatsu techniques, from basic finger pressure to more advanced stretches and joint rotations, catering to both beginners and seasoned practitioners. Through detailed explanations and visual aids, readers gain insight into the nuances of each technique, including the correct pressure, body mechanics, and timing required for effective application. The guide also emphasizes the importance of practitioner self-care, guiding users in maintaining balance and centering their energy to prevent burnout, which is essential for sustainable practice.

This book further illustrates the interconnectedness of physical, mental, and spiritual health by highlighting the role of breathwork, meditative awareness, and the therapeutic environment in maximizing Shiatsu's benefits. It empowers readers to integrate these techniques into daily self-care routines, fostering a deeper connection with their bodies and helping them address ailments at the root level.

By the end of the guide, readers are equipped with a versatile toolkit to address various health concerns, from stress relief and muscle tension to deeper emotional blocks. This book ultimately serves as a valuable resource that promotes a balanced, empowered approach to health, offering a pathway toward physical and emotional harmony through the healing power of touch.

THE END